Eyes

ALEKSANDER JEDROSZ

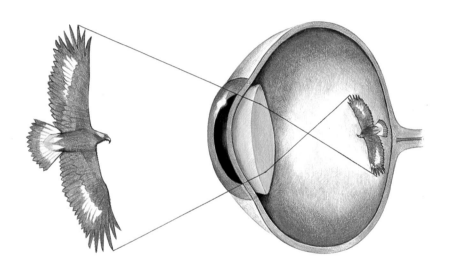

illustrated by
ANDREW FARMER and **ROBINA GREEN**

Troll Associates

Library of Congress Cataloging-in-Publication Data

Jedrosz, Aleksander.
 Eyes / by Aleksander Jedrosz; illustrated by Andrew Farmer &
Robina Green.
    p.   cm.
 Summary: Discusses the parts of the eye, how they function to
produce the phenomenon of vision in humans and animals, and other
aspects of the act of seeing.
 ISBN 0-8167-2094-0 (lib. bdg.)   ISBN 0-8167-2095-9 (pbk.)
 1. Eye—Juvenile literature.   2. Vision—Juvenile literature.
[1. Eye.   2. Vision.]   I. Farmer, Andrew, ill.   II. Green, Robina,
ill.   III. Title.
QP475.7.J43   1992
612.8´4—dc20   90-42177

Published by Troll Associates.

Edited by Neil Morris
Designed by COOPER-WILSON
Picture research by Jan Croot

Printed in the U.S.A.

10 9 8 7 6 5 4 3 2 1

Illustrators

Andrew Farmer front and back cover, pp 1, 2, 3,
 6-7, 7, 8, 9, 10, 10-11, 12, 13, 26
Robina Green front cover, pp 4, 5, 8, 11, 14, 16-17,
 20, 21, 23, 26, 27, 29
Additional illustrations by COOPER-WILSON

Picture credits:
Chris Fairclough 15
Science Photo Library (Ralph Eagle) front cover,
 (Jeremy Burgess) 5, (David Parker) 27,
 (Andrew McClenaghan) 28
John Watney 29

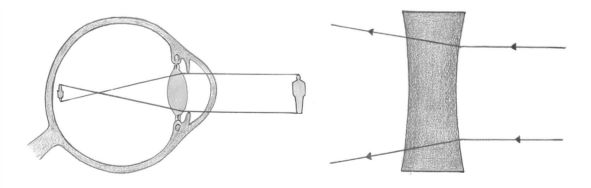

Contents

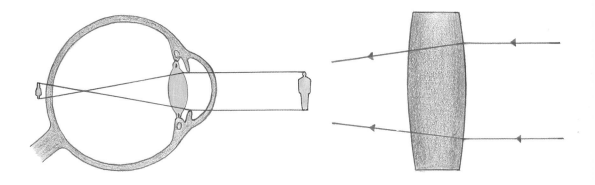

Eyes and senses

Things are happening around you all the time and your senses tell you all about them. You have five senses: your eyes see, your ears hear, your nose smells, your tongue tastes, and your skin feels.

Senses are your body's messengers, passing information along nerves in your body to your brain. Only when the brain has received the message are you aware of what you have tasted, seen, heard, smelled, or felt. Your senses work together, constantly reporting to your brain.

You rely on all your senses, but your eyes are the most important. It has been claimed that four-fifths of what we know reaches our brain through our eyes. However, we take our eyes for granted. Normally, we do not even think about them until something goes wrong with them.

▲ A crab's eyes are on short stalks that can move. This helps the crab look for food when hunting.

▲ Your eyes are very delicate. They are protected by eyelids and eyelashes, as well as eyebrows.

4

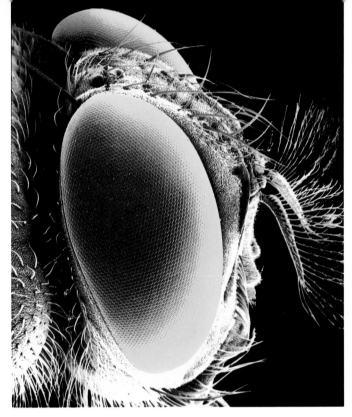

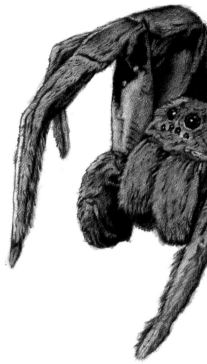

▲ Flies have compound eyes. These are like thousands of little eyes joined together, each pointing in a different direction. This means a fly can see all around it at the same time.

▲ Most spiders have eight eyes that help them look forward when catching food.

Our eyes react to light. Nearly all animals also respond to light, but their eyes vary as much as the animals themselves. If you look at an insect's eyes, you will see they are very different than ours. Birds can see colors as well as we do, but a cat probably sees only in black and white. Animals' eyes are designed for their particular needs, just as ours are.

Eyes do not just help you to learn. They also tell other people about you. Your eyes express emotions. Sometimes, if people want to hide their feelings, they hide their eyes. Your eyes are your windows on the world.

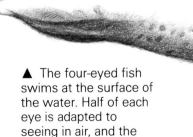

▲ The four-eyed fish swims at the surface of the water. Half of each eye is adapted to seeing in air, and the other half in water.

A look at your eye

Your eye is about the size of a table tennis ball, but you can only see the front. The rest of it is protected by the bony eye socket. Muscles let your eyes look up and down, and from side to side. But how do you actually see?

When it is pitch black, you see nothing. You can only see when there is light. As you look at this page, light from it reflects into your eye.

Letters on the page absorb all the light rays, so they appear black. Areas that reflect all the rays appear white. The colored areas absorb some parts of the light spectrum and reflect others, so you see different colors.

Many features of a camera are mechanical copies of what happens in the eye. First, light passes into the eye through a clear, protective shield called the *cornea.* Behind the cornea is the *iris,* which gives the eye its color. Muscles in the iris control the amount of light passing through a small opening in its center called the *pupil.*

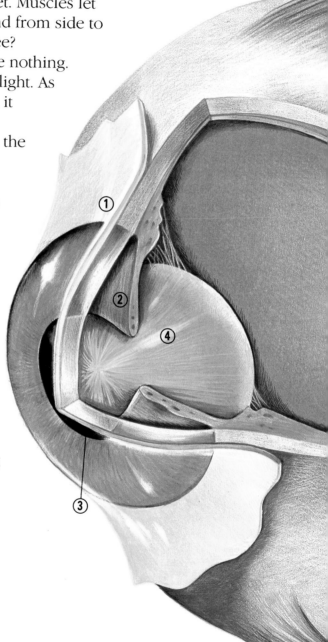

① cornea
② iris
③ pupil
④ lens
⑤ vitreous humor
⑥ retina
⑦ optic nerve

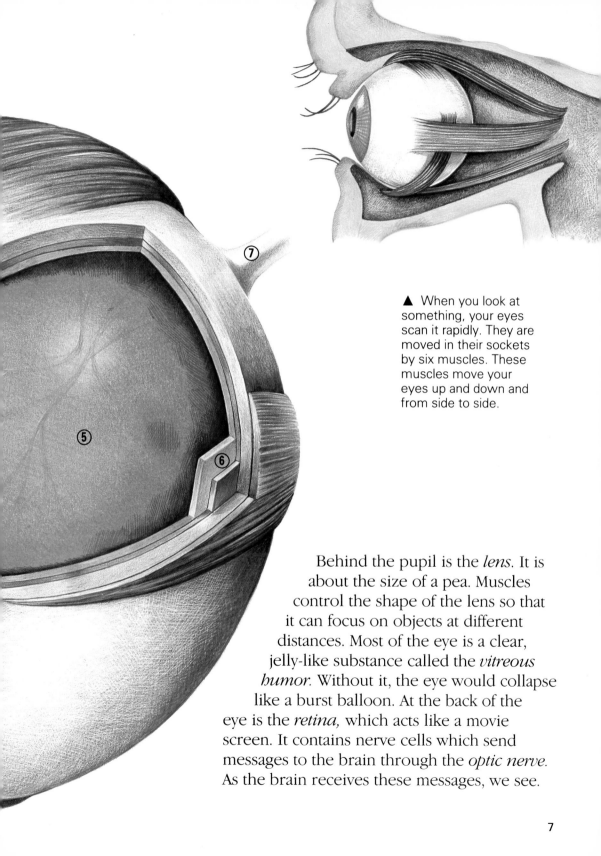

⑦

⑤

⑥

▲ When you look at something, your eyes scan it rapidly. They are moved in their sockets by six muscles. These muscles move your eyes up and down and from side to side.

Behind the pupil is the *lens*. It is about the size of a pea. Muscles control the shape of the lens so that it can focus on objects at different distances. Most of the eye is a clear, jelly-like substance called the *vitreous humor*. Without it, the eye would collapse like a burst balloon. At the back of the eye is the *retina,* which acts like a movie screen. It contains nerve cells which send messages to the brain through the *optic nerve.* As the brain receives these messages, we see.

How to focus

You are able to focus without thinking because your brain adjusts your eyes automatically. When you focus, your eyes swivel a little, the pupils change size and the lenses change shape.

Try this: get a friend to stand in front of you and look into your face. Measure the distance between your friend's pupils.

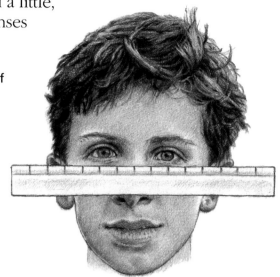

Now ask your friend to look out of the window at something. Measure the distance between his or her pupils again. The pupils should have been closer together in your first measurement. The closer an object is, the more your eyes swivel in to focus on it.

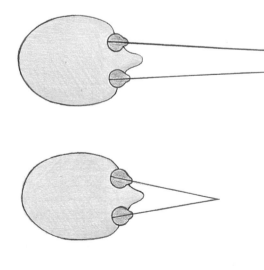

◄ Your eyes are constantly adjusting, responding to what you are looking at. The eye muscles make your eyes swivel in a little when you look at something close. Normally your eyes swivel only one sixteenth of an inch (one or two millimeters).

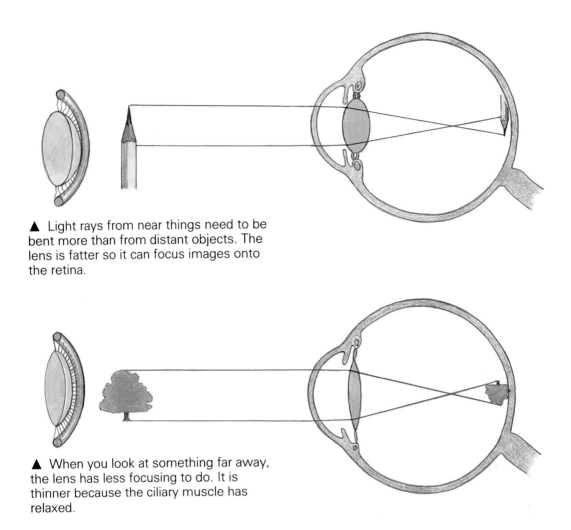

▲ Light rays from near things need to be bent more than from distant objects. The lens is fatter so it can focus images onto the retina.

▲ When you look at something far away, the lens has less focusing to do. It is thinner because the ciliary muscle has relaxed.

The lens is held in place by short threads called *suspensory ligaments,* and by a ring-shaped muscle called the *ciliary muscle.* This can change the shape of the lens. As the light rays pass through the eye, the cornea and the lens bend them toward each other. For us to see clearly, the rays must be focused onto the retina. When you look at something nearby, like the words on this page, the ciliary muscle contracts,

loosening the suspensory ligaments. These stop pulling the lens, so it gets thicker. Your pupils get smaller and your eyes swivel inward slightly.

When you look into the distance, the ciliary muscle relaxes. This causes the suspensory ligaments to tighten. These pull the lens, so it becomes flatter. Your eyes swivel out a little and your pupils become bigger.

How the retina works

An image of what you are looking at is focused on the retina, which contains about 126 million light-sensitive cells. These cells are divided into two types – *rod cells* and *cone cells.* They get their names from their shapes. The brain gets a constant stream of messages from the rods and cones. These messages are transmitted to the brain along the optic nerve.

Rod cells only make a black and white image, so they send black and white messages to the brain. The good thing about rods is that they need only a little light to work. Because there is so much light during the day, the rods are permanently activated. When you first enter a darkened room, you have difficulty seeing things. This is because it takes the rods a few minutes to become *dark-adapted.* Think about this the next time you go to the movies.

▼ The inner layer of the eye, the retina, is sensitive to light. The retina sends endless messages to the brain about what we see.

► The retina has millions of light-sensitive rod cells (**1**) and cone cells (**2**), which magnified would look like this.

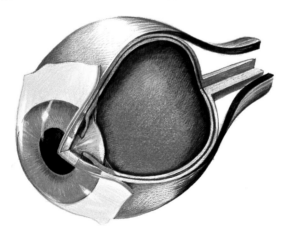

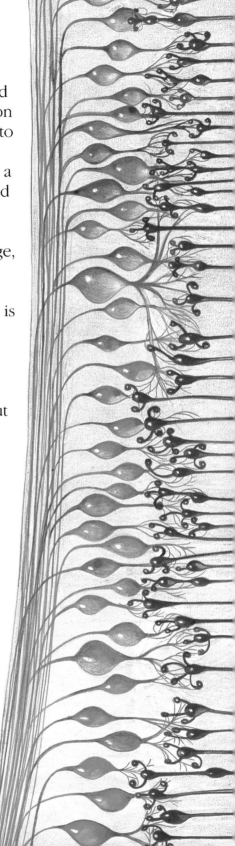

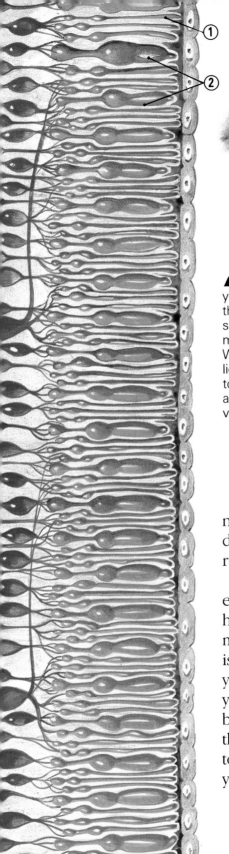

①

②

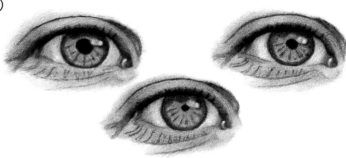

▲ The pupil is a hole in your iris. It lets light into the eye and can change size depending on how much light there is. When there is not much light, the pupil is large to let in as much light as possible. When it is very bright, the pupil is very small. Your pupils also change size according to your emotions. If you are excited, they get bigger, no matter what the light conditions are. When you look at something you do not like, your pupils contract a little.

Cone cells make a colored image, but they need lots of light to work. This is why it is difficult to see colors at night or in a dark room. There is just not enough light around.

Look at yourself in a mirror. If you close your eyes until they are almost shut, you will notice how your pupils get bigger. They are letting as much light as possible through the retina. This is what happens when you go out in the dark. If you now open your eyes quickly you will see your pupils shrinking. Because the light is bright, they are allowing less of it to get through to the retina. Your pupils work together. If you cover one eye with your hand, you will see the pupil of the other get larger.

Upside down and invisible

Your eye sees images upside down and backward. So does a camera.

Fortunately, you do not live in an upside-down and backward world. Your brain unscrambles what you see. A scientist once experimented with a pair of glasses which made him see things upside down and backward. After wearing them for a while, his brain corrected what he saw and he began to see things the right way! But when he removed the glasses, everything was upside down. Can you guess why?

▼ When you look at something, light from it is focused onto your retina. Light rays from the top of the object cross those from the bottom. This means that the image is upside down and backward on the retina. The image is corrected by the brain.

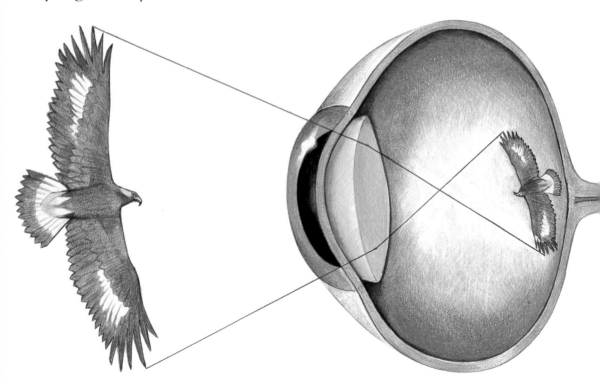

There are no rods or cones where the optic nerve leaves the eye, so this part of the retina is not sensitive to light. It is called the *blind spot*.

We do not normally experience these blind spots in everyday life. Our two eyes compensate for each other by overlapping their fields of vision.

▼ Optic nerves take messages from the retina to the brain. Nerves from the left side of the retina of both eyes go to the left side of the brain. Those from the right side of each retina go to the right side of the brain.

blind spot

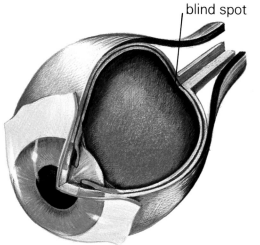

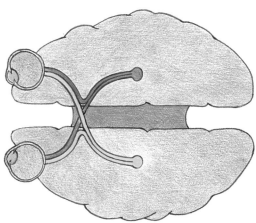

Try this: cover your right eye and look at the dog in the picture with your left eye. Hold the page about 6 inches (15 centimeters) away from you. Slowly move the book further away, but keep concentrating on the dog.

What happens to the ghost? You should find that it disappears and then reappears. When the image falls on your blind spot, the ghost vanishes. What do you have to do to make the dog vanish?

Two eyes are better than one

Have you ever asked yourself, "Why do I have two eyes?" Can you see twice as much with two, or is there another reason?

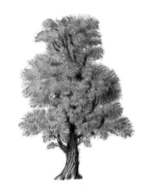

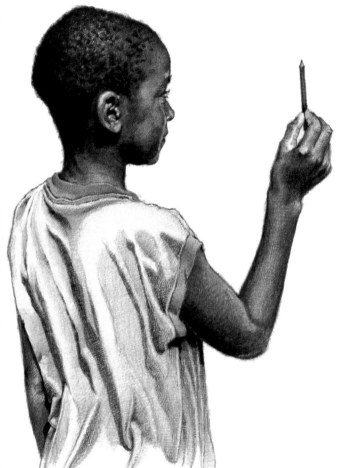

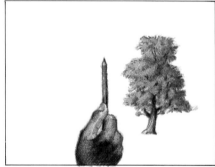

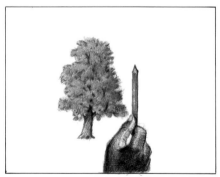

Try holding a pencil at arm's length. Line it up with a faraway object, such as a tree, putting the object between the two images of the pencil that you see. Close one eye. Now open your eye and close the other one. You should see that the pencil has "moved."

This happens because each eye makes a slightly different image of the scene you are looking at, so your brain is sent two different messages. It then puts the two images together, or *superimposes* them. It's a good thing that it does this — otherwise we would be seeing double all the time!

Now hold a pencil in each hand and bend your arms a little. Close one eye and quickly bring the pencils together so that their points touch.

Do it a few times. Then try it with both eyes open. Was it easier with one eye or two? You should have found that two eyes are better than one.

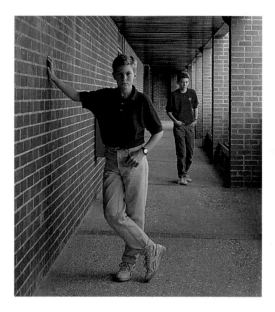

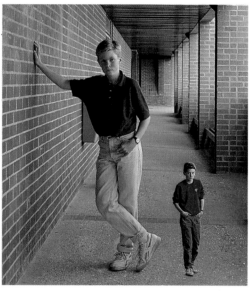

When you look at an object, your brain knows how much your eyes have swiveled in, or *converged*. The closer an object is, the greater the convergence must be for you to focus on it. However, this is not the only way you judge distance. An object can look large close up, but small if it is far away. This is called *perspective*. When we look at an object, its size helps to tell us how far away it is.

Our ability to merge the images received by each eye is called *stereoscopic vision*. This allows us to judge distance. It also makes objects seem solid, or three-dimensional, rather than flat. It helps us to see the world as it really is.

▲ The picture on the left shows us something that we expect to see: the boy leaning against the wall is larger because he is closer. In the right-hand picture something is wrong. The boy who is behind is now level with the boy leaning against the wall, but he is the same size as before. In this trick photograph the laws of perspective have been broken.

Field of vision

Have you ever thought about where your eyes are in your head? They face forward. But if you look at a rabbit's eyes, you will see that they are at the sides of its head. So it is not surprising that we see things differently from a rabbit. The rabbit's field of vision is much wider than ours.

Plant-eating animals, like rabbits and deer, are often hunted. To protect themselves, they have eyes on the sides of their heads. Each eye sees a completely separate area. Without moving its head, the animal can see what is in front, to the sides and even behind. But these animals have difficulty judging distance, because what one eye sees does not overlap much with what the other sees. Their vision is not stereoscopic.

▶ Hunters can judge distance very well because there is a great overlap between what each eye sees.

▼ Plant-eaters such as rabbits can see all around them without moving their heads. But they are not good at judging distance.

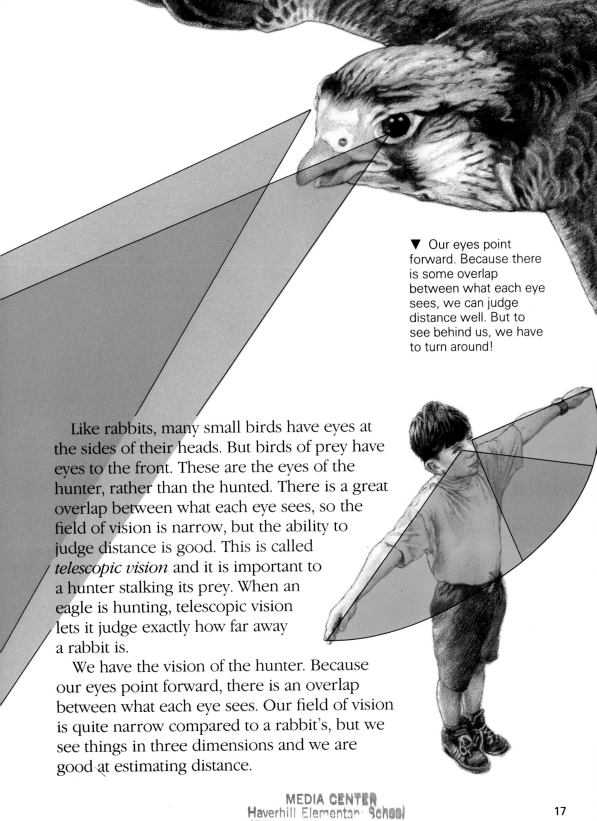

▼ Our eyes point forward. Because there is some overlap between what each eye sees, we can judge distance well. But to see behind us, we have to turn around!

Like rabbits, many small birds have eyes at the sides of their heads. But birds of prey have eyes to the front. These are the eyes of the hunter, rather than the hunted. There is a great overlap between what each eye sees, so the field of vision is narrow, but the ability to judge distance is good. This is called *telescopic vision* and it is important to a hunter stalking its prey. When an eagle is hunting, telescopic vision lets it judge exactly how far away a rabbit is.

We have the vision of the hunter. Because our eyes point forward, there is an overlap between what each eye sees. Our field of vision is quite narrow compared to a rabbit's, but we see things in three dimensions and we are good at estimating distance.

Seeing is believing – or is it?

An optical illusion is a picture which is not quite what it seems.

When you look at the picture below, do you see a vase or two people looking at each other?

What about this picture? Is it a young lady or an old woman?

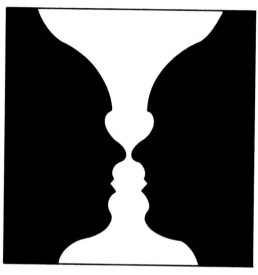

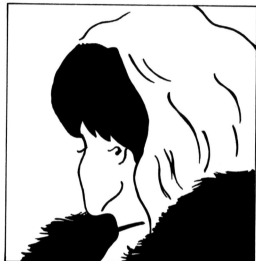

Sometimes when you glance at something, you are fooled because you expect to see something. It is only when you look more closely that you realize you have been tricked. What do you make of the following pictures?

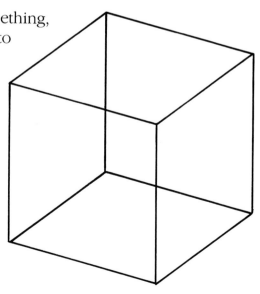

Here is a box. Are you looking down on it, or up at it?

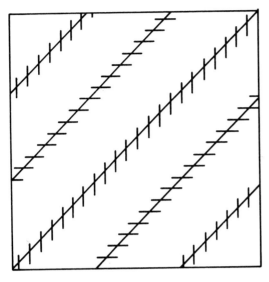

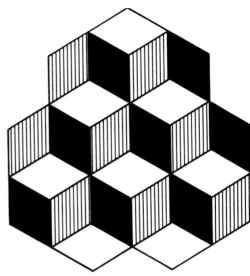

Are these five lines pointing in the same direction?

What about these cubes? How many are there? Can you see six or seven?

Which line is longer, A or B?

Which of these lines is longer, Y or Z?

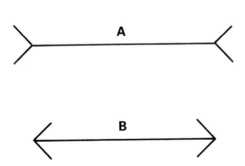

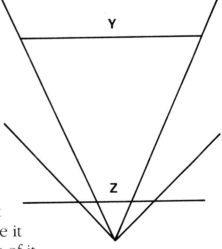

When you look at something, you want to understand it. No matter how strange it appears, your brain tries to make sense of it. Optical illusions test your ability to do this.

What color?

The world is full of color. Not all animals see in color, but we do. Artists use different colors to create a mood or to indicate feelings. They may use warm colors, like red or orange, to portray strong emotions or actions. A cool color, like green, can convey a peaceful feeling.

The effect of a color can be changed by surrounding it with different colors. The lightness or darkness of a color also changes the way we respond to it.

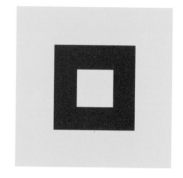

▲ Against a yellow background, the blue of the panel looks brilliant. This is because blue contrasts with yellow.

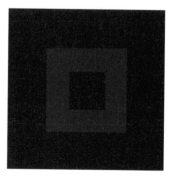

▲ Against a purple background, the same blue panel looks much paler. The blue is toned down by the deeper color.

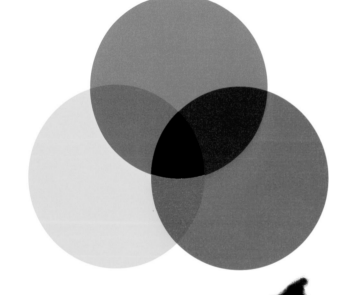

Blue, red, and yellow paint can combine to make any color. If they all overlap, black is produced.

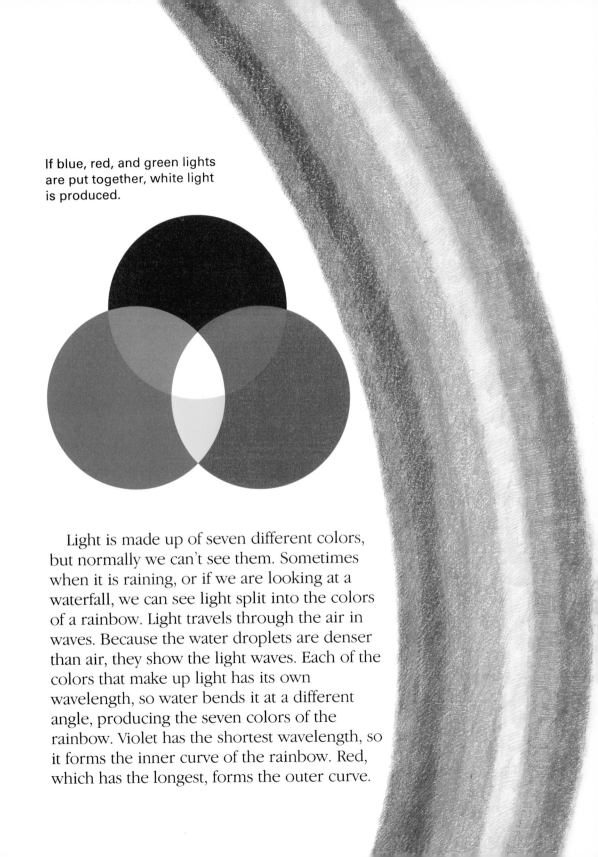

If blue, red, and green lights are put together, white light is produced.

Light is made up of seven different colors, but normally we can't see them. Sometimes when it is raining, or if we are looking at a waterfall, we can see light split into the colors of a rainbow. Light travels through the air in waves. Because the water droplets are denser than air, they show the light waves. Each of the colors that make up light has its own wavelength, so water bends it at a different angle, producing the seven colors of the rainbow. Violet has the shortest wavelength, so it forms the inner curve of the rainbow. Red, which has the longest, forms the outer curve.

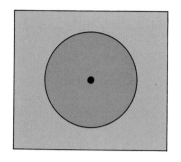 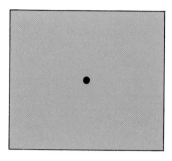 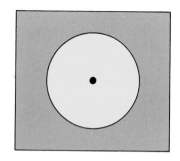

Try staring at the dot in the blue circle for about a minute. Now look at the dot in the gray square. What do you see? Now do the same with the yellow circle.

What do you see this time? Seeing one color after looking at another is called an *afterimage*. Usually we see the opposite, or complementary, color.

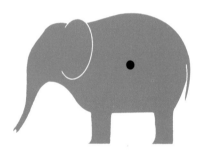

Stare at the spot in the middle of this green elephant for at least 30 seconds. Then look immediately at a white piece of paper. You should see a pink elephant!

Colors are paired in this way because color receptors in the eye are sensitive as pairs. When you stop looking at a color, that color is turned off and the other color in the receptor is turned on for a short time. Red and green are one complementary pair of colors, and purple and yellow are another pair.

If you look at the colored pictures in this book through a magnifying glass, you will see that they are made of lots of tiny dots. So are the colors on a TV screen. Your eyes and brain join the colored dots to make one image.

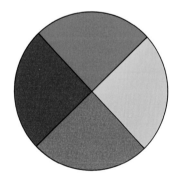

▲ Two pairs of complementary colors: red and green, and purple and yellow.

What color are your eyes?

The color of your iris is just one of the features you inherit from your parents. How does this happen?

You get some of your features from your mother and others from your father. These features, which include everything from the texture of your hair to the color of your eyes, are determined by *genes.* Genes are parts of cells that pass information from one generation to the next. Each feature is determined by combining one gene from your mother with one from your father. Some genes are stronger than other genes, and are most likely to dominate or *mask* them. If both of the genes that control eye color have "brown" information, then you will have brown eyes. If both genes have "blue" information, you will have blue eyes. But if one gene has "brown" information and the other has "blue," you will have brown eyes. The genes with "brown" information dominate the genes with "blue" information.

Is it possible for two brown-eyed parents to have a blue-eyed child? If both parents had one gene with "blue" information which had been masked by "brown" information, they could produce blue-eyed children.

These brown-eyed parents have a one in four chance of having a blue-eyed child. But it is unlikely that two blue-eyed parents would have brown-eyed children.

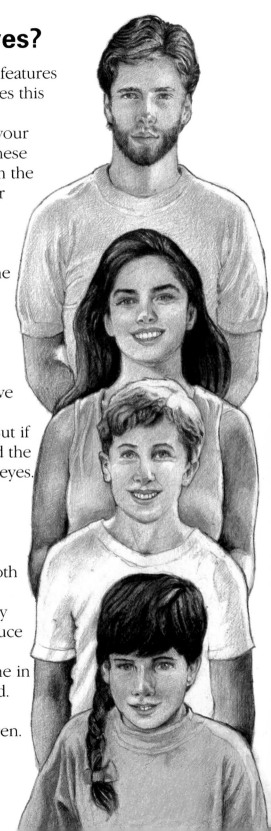

Are you colorblind?

Earlier in the book we discussed how the cone cells in our retina make colored images. Scientists think we have three types of color-sensitive cones. Some cones detect blue light, some green light, and some red light. When you look at something, different numbers of each type of cone are stimulated. Then your brain sorts out the colors that you see.

In Europe and America, about 7 percent of men have some form of what we call *color-blindness*. In females it is much rarer, affecting less than 1 percent. Colorblindness is generally passed down through the female side of families.

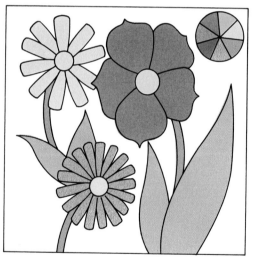 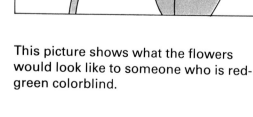

What colors do you see in this picture? If you see red, blue, and yellow flowers and green leaves, you are probably not colorblind. If you are not sure of the colors, you may be a member of a special group of people who are red-green colorblind.

This picture shows what the flowers would look like to someone who is red-green colorblind.

True colorblindness, which is very rare, is when a person sees only in black, gray, and white. This is called *achromatic vision.* It occurs only when the cone cells are missing, an inherited condition. Common colorblindness is not as serious, and people affected usually only have difficulty in telling the difference between greens and reds.

A colorblind person can often guess the color of an object from its shade. And while most of us look at the color of a traffic light, colorblind people look at the position of the light to tell them whether to stop or go. There is very little a colorblind person can't do.

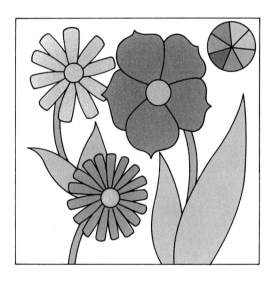

A few people may not be able to see blue and yellow, which would look like this.

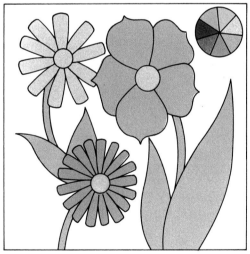

This picture shows what the flowers would look like to someone with achromatic vision.

Clearly being colorblind can be a problem where color differences are important. Can you think of some examples?

Things can go wrong

A healthy diet and good hygiene are your best defenses against eye complaints, but things can still go wrong.

It is common for people to lose their ability to focus properly. This usually happens because either the lens or the whole eye is the wrong shape. You are *nearsighted* if you cannot see distant things, and *farsighted* if you cannot see nearby things.

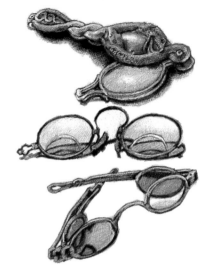

If you are nearsighted, light from faraway things is focused in front of the retina instead of on it. The cornea and the lens have bent the light in too much.

Glasses which bend the light out correct the problem. They have *concave* lenses, which are thinner at the center than around the edges.

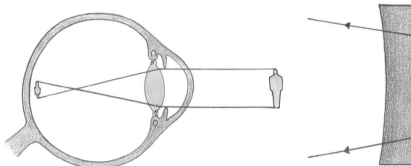

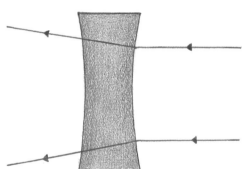

Farsighted people are unable to bend light rays in properly, so light focuses behind the retina instead of on it.

Glasses with *convex* lenses, which are thicker in the middle than around the edges, bend the light in.

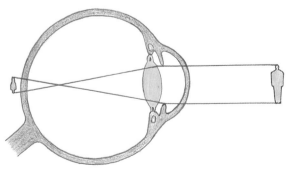

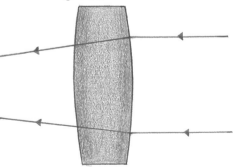

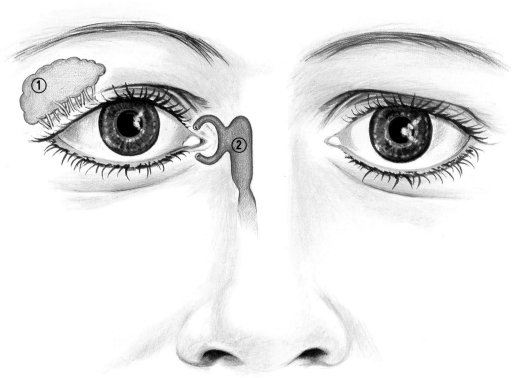

▲ Tears help keep the cornea moist. They flow from the lacrimal gland (**1**), drain through canals to the lacrimal sac (**2**), and into the nasal cavity.

▼ A contact lens is a small disk of thin plastic that fits over the cornea. Contact lenses correct vision in the same way as glasses.

As people get older, the cornea can mist over, or the lens may become cloudy. Both conditions keep light from getting to the retina, but they can be corrected by surgery. But a person with a replacement lens will still need glasses, because the new lens is plastic and cannot change shape like a human lens.

Minor problems that can affect our eyes are *sties* and *conjunctivitis.* A sty is an infection at the root of an eyelash. Conjunctivitis, which is sometimes called "pinkeye," irritates the lining of the eyelids and the eyeball. Both of these ailments are easily cured.

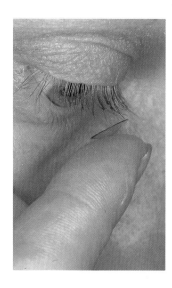

Healthy eyes

Because your eyes are so important, you must care for them properly. Here are some useful tips:

1 Have your eyes checked regularly by a doctor or an *ophthalmologist* (this is a medical doctor who is specially trained to look for eye disease).

2 When you are doing lots of close work, such as reading or writing, rest your eyes every half an hour or so by looking into the distance. This keeps your eyes from becoming tired.

3 Make sure you are in a well-lit place when you are doing close work. If you are right-handed, the light should come from over your left shoulder, and the other way around. This will allow you to see things without casting a shadow on them, which strains your eyes.

4 Avoid looking at bright lights and NEVER look at the sun through binoculars or a telescope. Remember, light activates the cells in the retina and too much light could damage the rods and cones permanently.

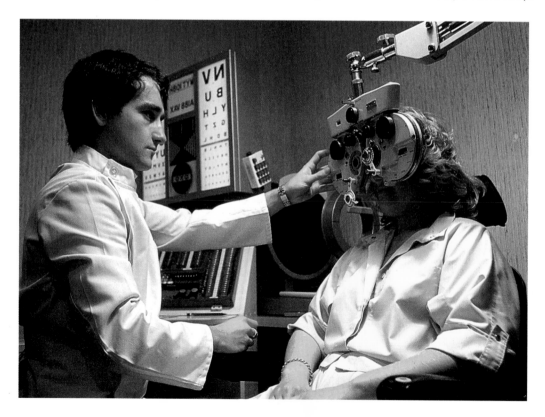

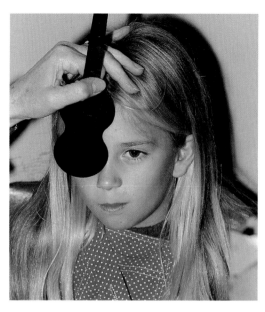

5 The rod cells in the retina need vitamin A to work properly. Foods that contain vitamin A include carrots, spinach, liver, and watercress. If you do not eat enough vitamin A, you will get "night blindness." This means that you will not be able to see very well in the dark.

6 Normally if we get dust in our eyes, it will be removed by our tears. Sometimes it helps to do some extra blinking. This will wash the eye out more quickly.

7 If you get an eye infection, go to the doctor at once.

▲ Everyone should have their eyes checked regularly.

◄ Here, a doctor checks a patient's eyesight with a special instrument. By turning knobs, different lenses are selected. The patient is looking through the lenses at a letter chart reflected in a mirror on the wall opposite.

► Working or playing on a computer is hard work for your eyes. As with other close work, you should rest your eyes regularly.

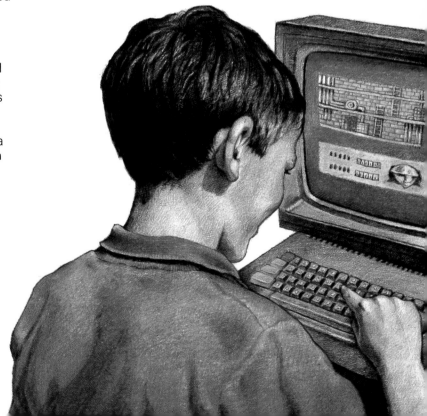

Glossary

achromatic vision a type of colorblindness when a person sees only in black, white, and shades of gray.

afterimage the image of something you still see when you look away from it.

blind spot part of the retina, where the optic nerve leaves the eye, that is not sensitive to light.

ciliary muscle a ring-shaped muscle that changes the shape of the eye's lens.

colorblindness an inherited inability to distinguish between certain colors.

concave a concave lens is thinner in the middle than around the edges and bends light out.

cone cells light-sensitive cells in the retina that let us see things in color, but only when there is enough light.

conjunctivitis inflammation of the conjunctiva, the delicate lining of the eyelids and eyeball.

convergence the degree of inward swing that results when your eyes look at something close.

convex a convex lens is thicker in the middle than around the edges and bends light in.

cornea the clear protective layer at the front of the eye, through which light passes.

dark-adapted rod cells become dark-adapted when you have been in the dark for a few minutes and you begin to see things that you could not see at first.

farsighted you are farsighted if you cannot see things that are near to you clearly.

genes parts of cells that pass information from one generation to the next, determining your features.

iris the colored part of the eye which surrounds the pupil and controls the amount of light entering the eye.

lens the transparent, elastic part of the eye just behind the iris that helps focus light onto the retina.

mask (of genes) to dominate or hide (other genes).

nearsighted you are nearsighted if you cannot see far-away things clearly.

ophthalmologist a medical doctor trained to test your eyes and treat eye disease.

optic nerve the nerve that carries messages from the eye to the brain.

perspective the appearance of objects according to how far away they are; they can look large close up, but small far away.

pupil the opening in the center of the iris that changes size according to the amount of light entering the eye.

retina the light-sensitive layer at the back of the eye where images are focused.

rod cells light-sensitive cells in the retina that respond only to black and white and work even when there is little light.

stereoscopic vision the ability to merge images from both eyes that gives depth to what we see.

sties (singular: **sty**) infections at the roots of eyelashes.

superimpose   to put (images) together.

suspensory ligaments   short threads that hold the eye's lens in place.

telescopic vision   the ability to judge far-away distances accurately.

vitreous humor   a clear jelly-like substance that fills most of the eye and gives it shape.

Index